# One Good Fall
## By
## David Farland

ISBN: 1492933503
ISBN-13: 978-1492933502

# Who Ben Was

At 16, Ben Wolverton was a straight-A student.

He's was a body builder and a natural athlete, standing 6 foot 4.

His favorite hobby was longboarding, and he even made videos of himself boarding and doing stunts.

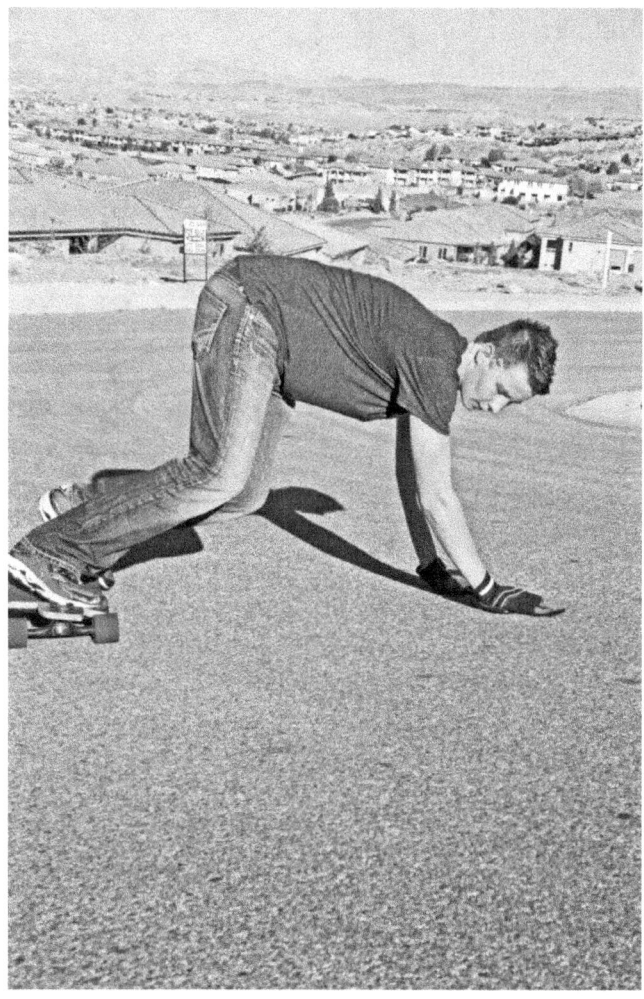

Here Ben is going down a hill, showing a stunt, without his helmet.

# Your First Good Fall May Be Your Last

As parents, we warned Ben repeatedly to always wear a helmet when he went longboarding. I told him over and over, "Your first good fall may be your last." On the rare occasions when we caught him without a helmet, we immediately grounded him.

But we had opposition. One of his friends had his own saying: "Helmets are for pussies."

On the afternoon of April 3, 2013, Ben asked to go longboarding with his friends. My last words to him that evening were, "Be sure to wear your helmet."

# An Unfamiliar Hill

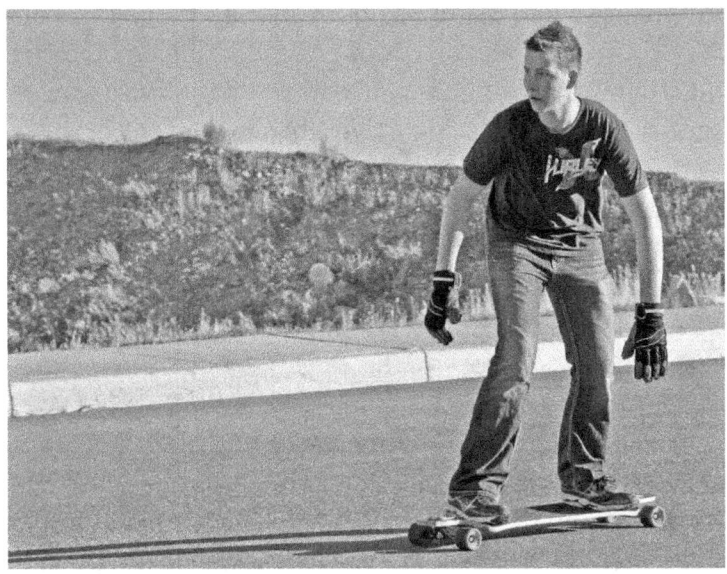

Ben and a friend went to a hill that they had never been down before.  It was steep.  On a hill like that, the board can easily hit 50 miles per hour.

Ben's friend went first, down a long slope and over a small rise, and found that his board began to wobble due to the high speed and uneven surface.  Once he was over the small rise, he turned to tell Ben not to come down, but he couldn't see Ben.

Suddenly a car pulled to a stop just over the hill, and the driver got out.  He shouted, "Your friend is down!"

# The Fall

Ben shattered the back of his skull, near the brain stem; the break was so bad that if you put your hands under his head and lifted, you could feel pieces of bone cracking and moving around. He also flipped end-over-end and got a concussion on the front-right side of his head, over the areas of the brain that deal with vision and speech.

The swelling on his brain caused both of his eardrums to break, and blood poured from them like a hose. It also poured from his nostrils. The policeman who first responded said, "I've never seen so much blood." Ben required several transfusions.

Ben broke vertebrae in his tail bone and also fractured both pelvis bones.

He bruised his lungs so badly that pneumonia set in within hours.

He scraped the skin from both knees, from his right shoulder, from his back, and part of his face, elbows, and fingers.

Ben was life-flighted 140 miles to the nearest hospital with a brain trauma unit.

Ben was such a mess, that we thought he would die, and we didn't want to remember him that way, so we didn't take any pictures.

# Ben's Brain Surgery

Twelve hours after Ben's accident, the pressure on his brain began to rise dangerously. This would cause the blood vessels to strangle, slowing the flow to the brain. Within hours the pressure could have killed him.

To relieve the pressure, the doctors asked to remove large parts of Ben's skull in a procedure called a "craniotomy."

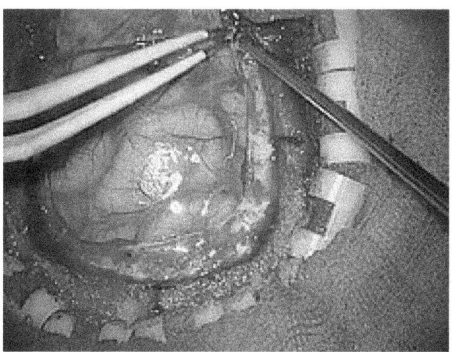

At one time I studied to be a doctor. Back when I was in pre-med, people who got a craniotomy only had a small chance of survival, about 15% in most hospitals. Survival rates are higher now, so long as the surgery is performed in time.

We only hoped that Ben would survive.

# The Wait Begins

Just after Ben's brain surgery, we asked the doctors about his chances.

The surgeon said, "We're just hoping that we can keep him alive for the next fifteen minutes, and then we'll worry about the fifteen minutes after that. If he lives for four days, the swelling in his brain should begin to go down. But even that doesn't guarantee that he will survive. Last month I told some parents that their son was out of the woods, eleven days after his accident, and he died thirty minutes later. I won't make that mistake again. I don't want to give you false hopes. We won't really know for weeks."

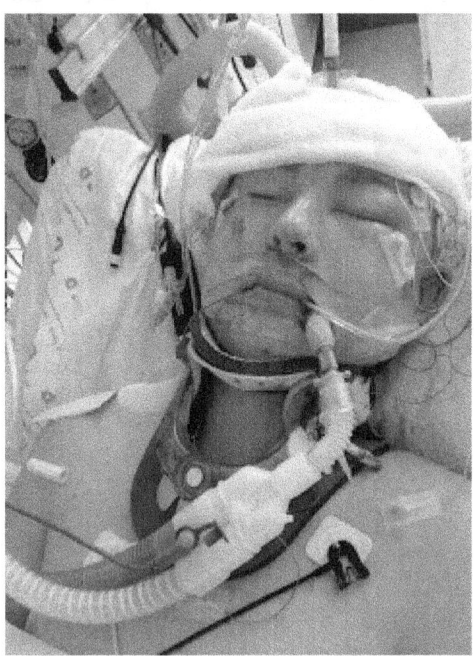

Ben in his coma, 11 days after the accident.

# Animal, Vegetable, or Mineral?

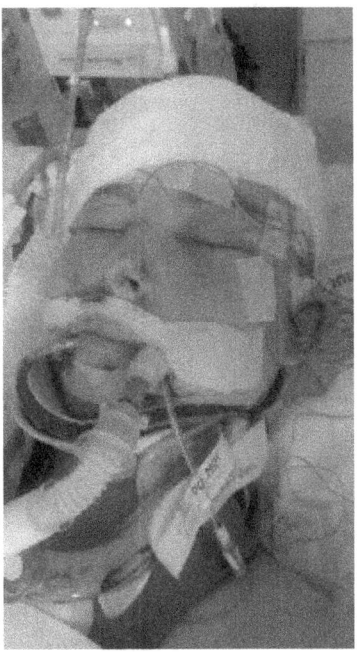

This is what Ben looked like after he got cleaned up from his craniotomy. It's the first picture we took after his accident.

He had both sides of his skull removed, and a narrow strip of bone was left down the middle of his head. The doctors cut open Ben's stomach and inserted the bones from his skull under the skin for safe storage, so that they could put them in later.

He got 80 staples in his head when they closed the wound there, and another 80 in his stomach.

It took several days for the blood to stop flowing from his ears.

Ben was put on a respirator to help him breathe.

He had a hole drilled in his head, and an instrument that looks like a meat thermometer was inserted into his skull to check the pressure of the fluid on his brain.

Ben was fed by a tube through his nose, and he drank from his IV's in each arm and in his leg.

He was put on antibiotics because he had a severe case of pneumonia, and he frequently had to have the doctors drain fluid from his lungs. When that happened, he would sometimes cough violently and throw up.

After three days without seeing Ben move, I remembered the old guessing game that starts with the guessers asking the question, "Animal, Vegetable, or Mineral." I looked at Ben and decided, "Definitely vegetable."

# We Spent Weeks Praying

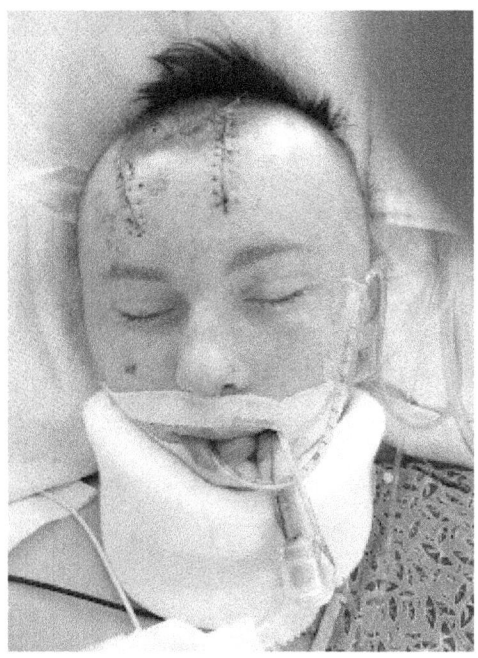

Ben didn't move for days, other than when the respirator helped him breathe.  The doctors monitored his brain pressure, brain activity, blood pressure, heart rate, and so on.

They didn't give us much hope.  We asked if he would recover, and one nurse said, "What you see is what you've got.  No one can say for sure if he'll even breathe on his own."

All that we could do for him really was pray, and thousands of people around the world joined in.  We heard from old friends in Japan, strangers in Samoa, business associates from Germany, and fans of my writing from South Africa, Australia, England, Malaysia, India, Russia, and many other countries.  Everyone lent emotional support.

When Ben finally did move, he started with his left leg, but only kicked.   After ten days, he squeezed his mother's hand, but the nurse said, "That doesn't mean anything.  It's the same reflex that a baby has."  But to his parents, it did mean something: at least Ben could move.

# The Bills Mount

As Ben's Dad I write for a living. Because I have diabetes, in the state of Utah I was unable to buy health insurance. None of the carriers in the state would cover me at all, nor would they cover my wife's pre-existing problems. So when the accident happened, my wife and I were searching for a job that would let us get on a group policy.

As a result, our family gets to cover all of the bills.

The life flight alone cost over $30,000. Radiologists, blood transfusions, and so on in the first hour cost thousands more. On day 14, I asked the hospital how much we owed. The bill at that time was $470,000 for the hospital. That didn't count the neurosurgeons, radiologists, pediatricians, and so on.

Our family was already over half a million dollars in debt, and Ben hadn't even opened his eyes.

# Ben Begins to Waken

Ben didn't move or speak for a long time.  When he did move, it started with his left leg, then his left arm.  He thrashed around a bit, but didn't groan or speak.

After a couple weeks he could squeeze his left hand, just a little, but his right side was too damaged.

We began to exercise him, and on a few rare occasions he would kick his left leg and seemed to help with his stretches.  I would say "Lift your left leg," and Ben would do it, sometimes.  Then I would say, "Now push!"

But Ben couldn't always do as asked.  Sometimes he would go three or four days without showing any sign of consciousness.

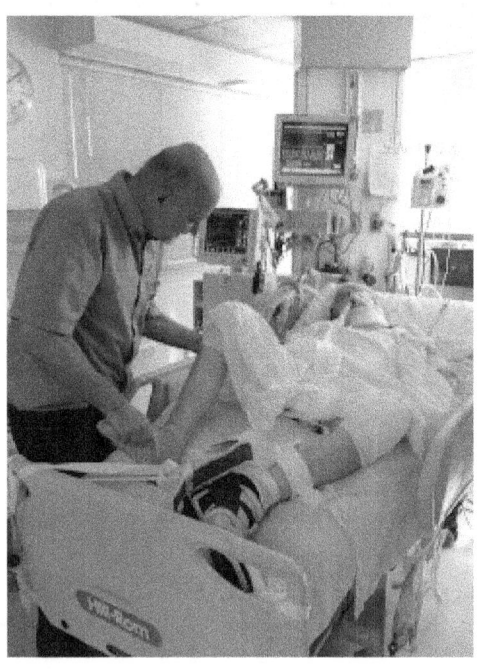

# After 15 Days Ben Opened His Eyes

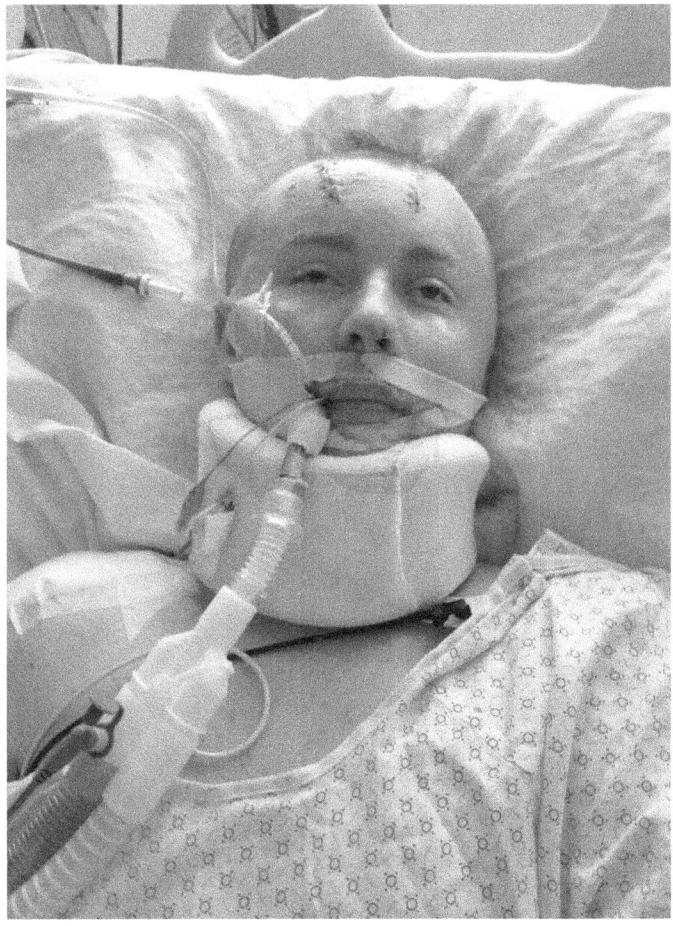

Ben began to open his eyes, and everyone was happy for that. He soon began to move his right hand and right leg. He moved his neck, and we were happy that it looked as if he would have some mobility, but he still wasn't conscious.

He couldn't talk, didn't recognize anyone. He didn't know where he was or what had happened. He was in terrible pain.

At this point, the most that he could do was rip the feeding tubes and breathing tubes out of his mouth and nose, and sometimes he would take a punch at a nurse.

So the nurses tied his arms and legs to the bed.  He soon began to get scrapes on his wrists, ankles, and feet from his incessant struggling.  When he fought too hard, the nurses would sedate him, sometimes with drugs strong enough to put him back into a coma.  This happened every day.

Still, he was getting better.

# Then Ben Got Really Sick

After a month, Ben's pneumonia grew worse, and he fell into unconsciousness. When the doctors came on their morning rounds, they avoided his parents and wouldn't answer questions. Instead they huddled near workstations, far from Ben's room.

Ben's fever rose to 105 degrees Fahrenheit. His white blood cell count rose, too. The doctors induced another coma and put him on a refrigerated bed to bring his temperature down, while we tried cooling his skin with ice cubes. His lips became terribly chapped and swollen.

Ben developed terrible diaper rash and bedsores.

The doctors kept changing his medications, taking samples of fluid from his lungs, and trying to fight his infections. But it was a losing battle. Ben was constantly coughing up blood and vomiting.

After nearly four weeks, we had thousands of people following Ben's "progress" on Facebook, but I realized that, most likely, by the next day he would have to tell them that Ben had finally died.

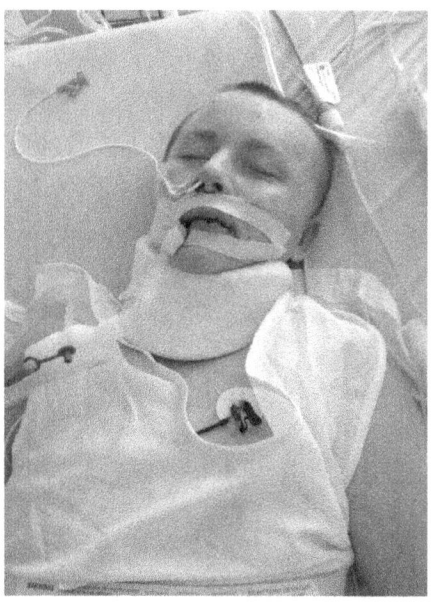

# The Misshapen Head

When Ben had his craniotomy, the doctor said that as soon as the skull cap was removed, Ben's swollen brain would shove its way about an inch above the line of the skull. So for weeks his head was over-large, and it made him look deformed.

If you touched his head where the skull had been removed, it felt a little like Jello. When Ben moved, his brain jiggled.

Then the swelling receded, and his skull suddenly caved-in, leaving big dents in his temples.

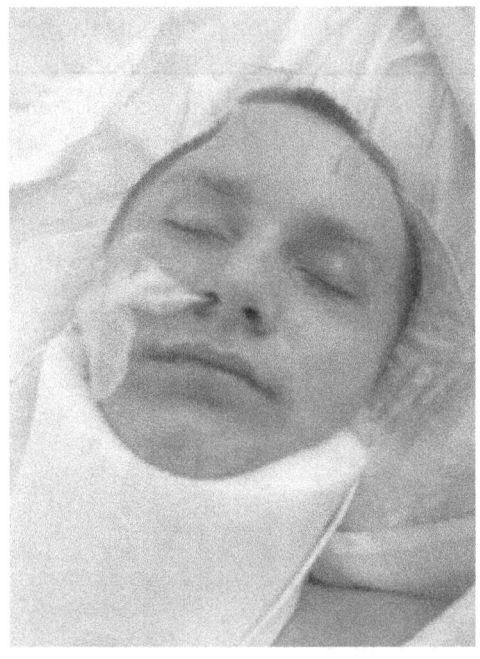

# Ben Wakes Up

Suddenly, more than a month after his accident, Ben woke up. The first thing that Ben recalls after the accident is talking to his older brother, Spencer.

When Spencer told Ben that he had fallen from his longboard, Ben didn't believe it. When Spencer pointed out that Ben had his skull in his stomach, and that it was proof of the fall, Ben said, "Hunh-uh, that's my six-pack. I've been working out."

Ben had not been able to do anything but groan or grunt for the previous weeks, but now he began to whisper. He was groggy, fading in and out. His throat was sore from all of the breathing tubes and feeding tubes in it. He could smile if we asked him to, and nod, but mostly he was hungry.

The doctors wouldn't let him eat or drink until he could prove that he could swallow, and Ben wasn't ready to do that. Nor could he walk, or even sit up by himself. We were able to sit him up, but only if he wore a special helmet.

Ben's mom pointed out the irony of it: Ben hadn't wanted to look stupid for 30 minutes while he was skating, but now he got to look stupid for the next sixty days. He couldn't even get out of bed without a helmet.

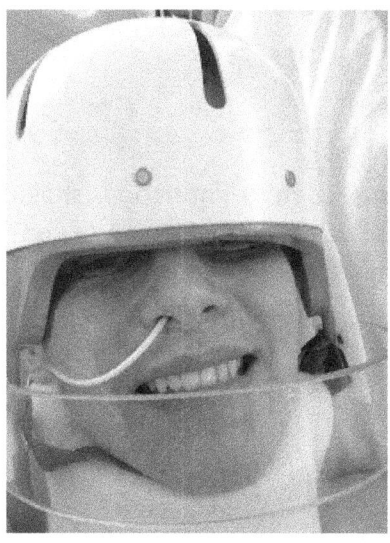

# Ben's Diet

Ben lost nearly fifty pounds while he was in the hospital. After he woke, he wasn't able to begin eating for days, until he could pass a "swallow test." He tried to drink, but that got fluid into his lungs, which gave him pneumonia again. Since he couldn't swallow properly, he continued to be fed a diet of "thickened liquids." It took another month before he was allowed to drink.

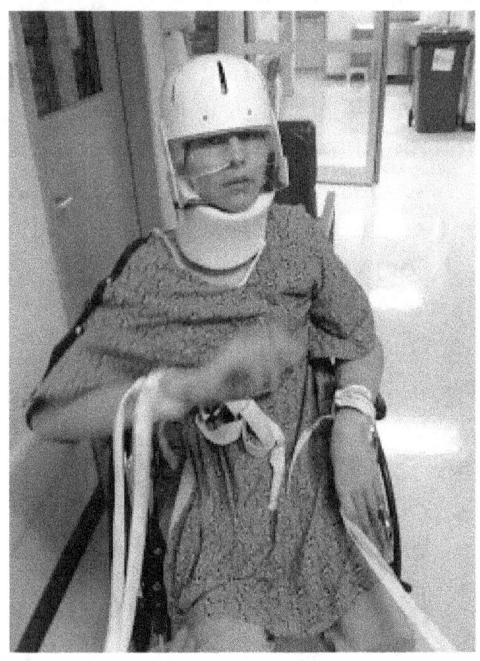

(In this picture, Ben's right hand is shaking uncontrollably due to tremors. This lasted for weeks. We kept him from having seizures by using medication.)

# Getting Around

Five weeks after the accident, Ben was ready to try his first steps.

Mostly, orderlies carried him by grabbing his arms and lifting, and then Ben tried to move his legs so that he "sort of" walked. His right side was too weak to bear much weight, and even his head hung to the side.

Still, he began to recover, making progress every day.

Ben was lucky. Many kids in similar situations aren't able to get up and walk for a year or more—if they ever do get out of bed again.

We think that much of Ben's quick recovery had to do with his natural athleticism. Even after a month in bed, his muscles were surprisingly firm. Having a thick skull might have helped, too.

Ben's doctors called his recovery "miraculous."

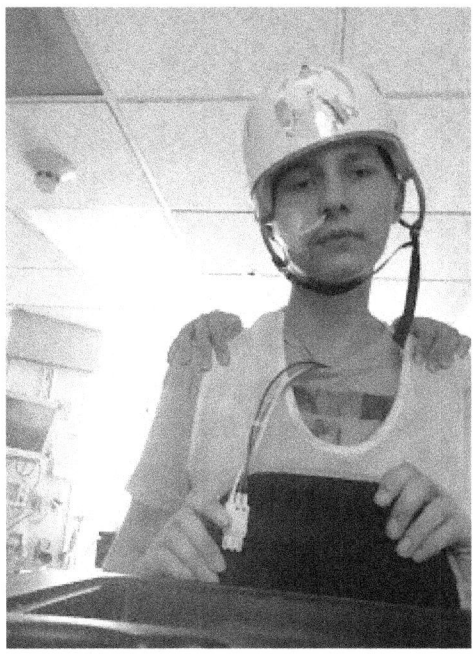

(Ben walks on a treadmill.)

# Brain Trauma Is Embarrassing

Ben ran into problems that we didn't expect. When Ben got transferred from one hospital to another, we found that he had lost so much weight, his pants kept falling down.

He was too weak to stand, and too uncoordinated to do two things at the same time. So his pants fell down and he tripped—several times.

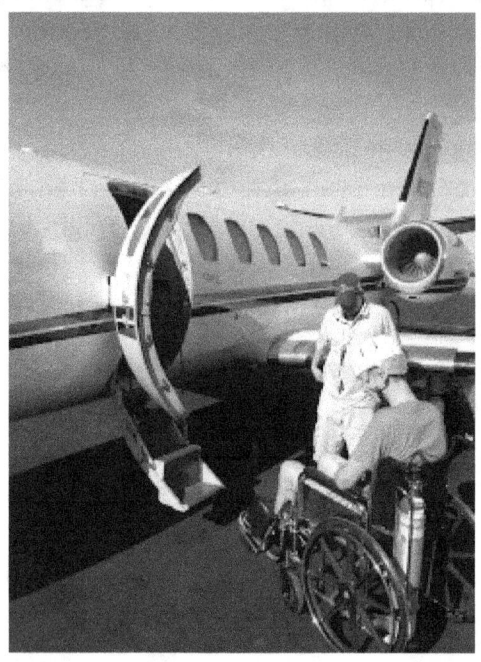

We heard dozens of embarrassing anecdotes from other brain trauma patients. Sometimes they become confused. One man recalled screaming in terror because he thought that his parents were giant praying mantises, trying to eat him.

Some people forget important information. One man wrote and told how he had forgotten how to speak English, and only remembered how to speak a little German that he had learned in high school.

# The Recovery Isn't Over

Brain trauma victims have a lot of problems. Sometimes things just get scrambled up. When Ben's speech therapist asked Ben what he had for lunch, Ben answered, "Potatoes, and peas, and kachuma."

"What's kachuma?" the therapist asked. Ben couldn't describe it. (It was chicken cordon bleu.)

Many easy mental tasks became challenging. Ben had a hard time figuring out how to put things in order. For example, in describing how to make a hamburger, Ben thought that you should eat it, then put on the bun, then fry it, and put on ketchup.

The biggest problem now, after six months, is called "brain fatigue." Mental stimulation can cause Ben to become tired. So, after watching a movie he may need to sleep. But physical stimulation can be just as exhausting. Taking a walk doesn't tire his muscles, but may be hard to handle mentally.

Ben is going to school, but needs to take a reduced load for at least the coming year. No more honors classes for him. Cognitive tests show that mentally he is now four or five years behind where he was last year. In addition to anti-seizure medicines, Ben is also being treated for depression, and being tested for other disorders.

It will be a struggle, doctors think that he will recover, more or less. He'll always be a few IQ points shy of where he was.

What's more surprising is what he *can* do. For example, Ben could hardly walk after his accident, but he could still play the guitar.

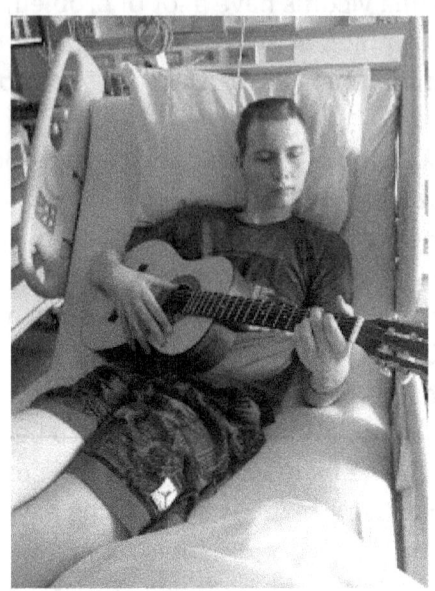

## What Did We Learn?

If you suffer a traumatic brain injury, everything that happened to Ben will probably happen to you--the surgeries, the coma, the pneumonia, the diaper rash, the disfigured face, the scars, the depression, the mental struggles.

You will never completely recover from the accident, either physically, emotionally, or financially.

# Action Items

—Pass this book around to children and teens who are mature enough to view it.

—If you personally don't wear a helmet while skateboarding, biking, or driving your motorcycle or ATV, start doing it now.  Encourage your friends to do the same.

You can find a huge selection of helmets if you look online.  For example, there is a wide selection at zappos.com/skateboard-helmet-helmets-pads.  Once you find a helmet, decorate it!  You can find very cool stickers, decals, and wraps online that will let you personalize your helmet and make it unique.  You can even make humorous helmets!

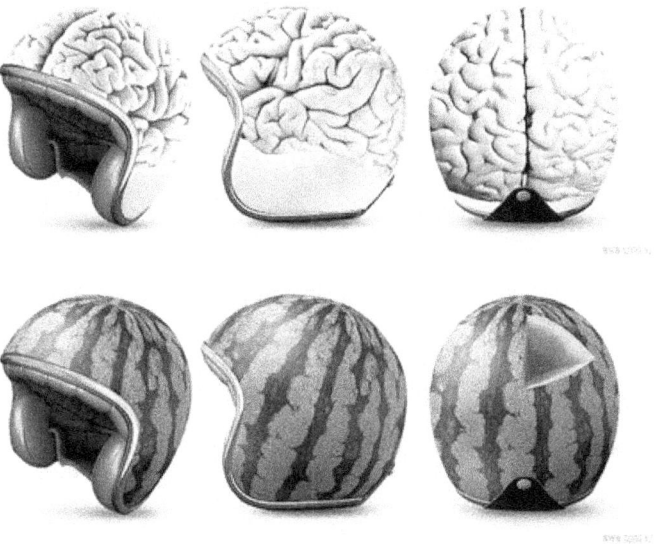

—If your community doesn't have laws against skateboarding or biking without a helmet, sponsor a new law.

—If you see a child biking or boarding without a helmet, do him a favor and report him to the police. You just might save a life. After all, would you really want someone that you care about to go through this?

# Ben's Happy Ending

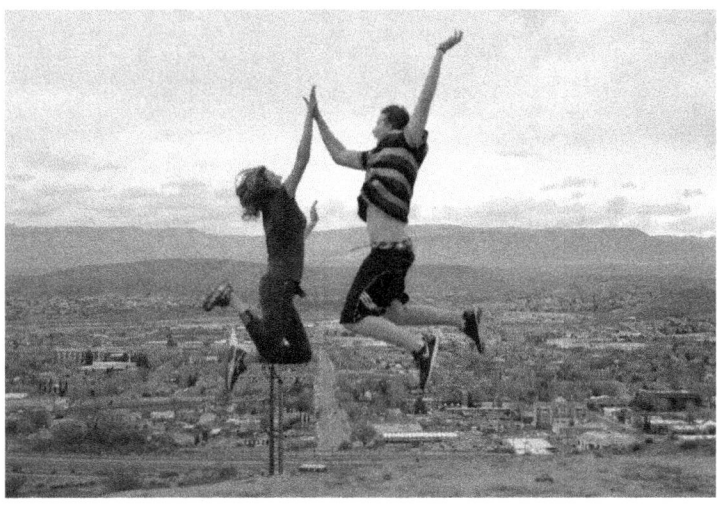

Here is Ben with his sister a few days before the accident. We hope to see him like this again someday. . . .